GINGER AND ITS MEDICINAL USES

GINGER AND ITS MEDICINAL USES

Compiled and Edited
by
Christopher N Burchett

PILGRIMS PUBLISHING
◆ Varanasi ◆

GINGER AND ITS MEDICINAL USES

Compiled and Edited by

Christopher N Burchett

Published by:
PILGRIMS PUBLISHING

An imprint of:
PILGRIMS BOOK HOUSE
(Distributors in India)
B 27/98 A-8, Nawabganj Road
Durga Kund, Varanasi-221010, India
Tel: 91-542- 2314060,
Fax: 91-542- 2312456
E-mail: pilgrims@satyam.net.in
Website: www.pilgrimsbooks.com

Layout & Cover design by Asha Mishra

ISBN: 81-7769-621-1

Printed in India at Pilgrim Press Pvt. Ltd. Lalpur Varanasi

GINGER

The use of and the practice of prescribing herbal and natural medicines have been in existence since time immemorial. Man has from his very inception looked to his surroundings for cures from his everyday ills. Fortunately nature has always provided us with plants, herbs and minerals that aid us in overcoming disease. In fact the whole system within which we exist appears to have been designed to provide us with food sustenance and certain medicinal plants to counteract the more destructive forces that exist within the whole scheme.

Recent studies of the genome have no doubt led scientists to believe that they have found the basic formula for the construction of living forms and thus the claims of the genetic engineers to be able to produce life forms that will be almost indestructible do not seem too far away. Unfortunately the vast majority, whilst rejoicing at this promise of an almost disease free society have neglected to refer back to the causes of many of the life taking diseases.

When looked at rationally it becomes apparent that man is, in fact, his greatest enemy, for many of the causes of disease may be traced to his abuse of and mismanagement of nature and his natural environment. Many of the diseases that we are forced to face are the results of overcrowding and unsanitary conditions that we ourselves have found necessary to create in our search for advancement and better living standards.

It was the move from nature to live in the crowded environs of the cities, where it may be noted that the 'haves' created much better living conditions for themselves than those created for the 'have-nots'. It was these overcrowded and unhygienic conditions that led to the spread of the more destructive and contagious diseases. As man adapted himself to these new living conditions far away from the open fields and fresh air of rural existence, so he managed to build up a resistance to some of these ailments. But when his brethren from the villages came into contact with this new life, they having no inbuilt resistance to these new diseases often fell foul to their embrace.

It may be safely said, therefore, that in many respects mankind in his search for supremacy over his environment has been the prime mover in his own downfall. Medical science may have reduced infant mortality only to create the greater enemy of overpopulation. Scientists have extended the period of life expectancy only to produce an even larger number of old age pensioners who no longer are able to actively take part in the upkeep of the society that they have produced. There are so many examples of man and his folly that it would be enough to fill a book on its own.

The purpose of this small volume is not to criticize or complain but rather to provide an ailing society with an alternative that may be used more as a prevention than as a cure. The hope that may be somewhere a spark of common sense still lives and that all men whether rich or poor, may once more think over their life styles and consider a more suitable and congenial way of existence, living in harmony with all around. To adopt a life that takes only from nature what it really needs and that is truly beneficial to it.

MEDICINE THOUGH THE AGES

When we talk about ancient or Oriental medicines or medical systems as a whole we are compelled to first of all understand their conceptual backgrounds. Looking back several thousands of years from the twenty-first century one would quite reasonably assume that the basic approach applied in these systems has become very much outdated and obsolete, especially when we consider the apparent advances made in modern medical science. These advances, real or imaginary, and when compared with the state of medicine only a few hundred years ago would support the assumption held of the primitiveness of these systems. Theories and hypotheses held then about such subjects as anatomy and the functions of certain organs have been disproved time and time again. But this is also true in many fields and in fact certain more modern theories and suppositions have also been thrown out of the window by even more recent and more comprehensive theories.

But this parochial approach to the subject completely overlooks many of its broader aspects. To completely reject systems that have survived for centuries and that have and still do bring relief to millions, out of hand, on the basis of conjectures made by more recent experts in the field would not be completely fair. It would be less so if one were to realise that these latest views have simply developed out of a new approach to these ancient systems. For example, the extreme interest being taken in the herbs of the Amazon rain forests and their medicinal values are but tip of the iceberg. If one were to realise that many so-called new medicines are in fact refined versions of more traditional medicines, penicillin being a prime example, then the efficacy of many potions created from these herbs would be of more general interest.

The ancient Egyptians, Greeks, Indians, Chinese and Japanese all had developed medical systems. Much of our knowledge of these systems has come from well-documented texts and not from hearsay as we have been led to believe. In fact if looked at closely we shall find that the basis of modern biomedicine has its roots in these systems. It is true that the lack of technology available to these systems in certain fields did not allow them to have the sophisticated instruments of the modern age, but this certainly did not decry their identification of certain ailments and their causes. In fact this lack of technology may have enabled them to develop certain other skills that modern doctors no longer possess. To illustrate this we should mention the capacity to identify the source of an illness through the pulse alone as being one, example identification of an ailment by observation alone being another and so on. Though apparently very hit and miss methods, it is surprising how successful they were in curing the sick and infirm. There are examples too where superstition plays a great role in identifying ailments and this still does exist in some parts of the world. It is for such afflictions that certain societies employ the services of shamans and exorcists to chase away the devils that have possessed their loved ones.

The ancient systems have to be divided into two distinct groups, the Indo-European and the Sino-Japanese. The Indo-European group includes the Egyptian, Greek and Ayurvedic systems and the Sino-Japanese the Korean, Chinese, Japanese and to some extent the Tibetan systems. Though it should be noted that the Tibetan system is more of a synthesis of Ayurveda, Chinese medicine and the Bon-Po shamanistic practices, which places it slightly apart from all the others.

The main concern evoked by all of these was the internal harmony within the human body itself. Each of the systems had accepted that the human body consisted of not only the physical frame but that it also relied upon its spirit as its main driving force. The harmony between the body and the spirit was, as far as they were concerned, essential for a healthy and trouble free life. So whether it is called '*prana*', '*ki*', '*qi*', '*ruh*' or spirit all the schools agreed on the most basic principle that health itself required a conscious attempt on the part of each individual to maintain an equilibrium between themselves and their environment—something forgotten by more modern man in his quest to conquer and rule the elements around him.

As in all ancient cultures the use of herbs in Western society was a common feature in the treatment of all ailments. The differing climates may have produced separate diseases and the herbs used may not have been so exotic but still there were medicines commonly administered in the home long before the inception of an organised medical profession. These remedies were generally well known amongst the common folk and provided respite from ailments that afflicted the people. These remedies, of course, varied from place to place but invariably the results were the same.

Ancient Egypt, the home of the pyramids, has been thought by many to have played a pivotal role in the development of the early western civilisations and much of the Greek knowledge found its source in the developments that took place in the earlier Egyptian society. Even today scientists search for the true secrets of the science behind the construction of the Pyramids. Papyrus records, from as far back as 4500 in the pre Christian era, tell us of the use of balsam, perfumed oils, scented barks and resins and the production of aromatic vinegars, wines and beer. The specific formulations were blended by priests, who at the same time interpreted the will of the Gods for the people, whilst performing the duties of physicians. They recorded their recipes for illness, for restoring youthfulness, for hay fever and for contraception.

Through archaeological studies we have come to know that their temples served not only as houses of worship but as laboratories as well. They imported their herbs from as far afield as India, China, Somalia and Malaysia. Frankincense and myrrh of Biblical fame, caraway and anise, barks of the cedar-wood and cypress were a few of the many herbs and plants that they employed. The priests used hundreds of pounds of these herbs to make the aromatic oils that they used to burn in the temples. They anointed their gods with these oils, a specific oil for each god (artemisia for Isis, marjoram for Osiris etc.). The Egyptians believed that the mortal body was equally important in the after-life as it was in the mortal world and they discovered that the aromatic oils that they had developed had preservative effects. Thus the art of embalming the dead developed and each embalmer developed his own secret formula, which was an understandably closely deguarded secret. This process also entailed a detailed knowledge of the physiology of the human body, as vital organs were removed before this process began and stored in a solution of sodium carbonate. Once this had been done, the body was bathed in essential oils and soaked in aromatic resins. After three months, the body was then wrapped in a gauze cloth that had been impregnated with resin, usually cedar wood and myrrh. This whole process took anything up to six months to complete, but much depended on the status of the person to be embalmed, royalty taking up much more time than the common man. This system proved so successful that even in the present day we have examples of almost perfectly preserved intestines almost 3000 years old. It is said that some of the earliest mummies found were transported back to England and France, where their gauze wrappings were soaked in alcohol and the resultant liquid that was strained off was sold as a medicine to increase the resistance to disease.

The ordinary Egyptians used these aromatic herbs in their cuisine as a digestion promoter thus showing their knowledge of the true properties of these herbs as well as their understanding of their medicinal qualities. It is rumoured that it was not Cleopatra's beauty alone that won the favours of the Roman General Mark Antony, but her knowledge and use of exotic perfumes that truly won his heart.

With the expansion of the Roman Empire into Northern Europe they carried with them many varieties of herbs that they commonly used as well as bringing the more sophisticated information gained from Greek and Egyptian sources, further knowledge became available and a primitive medical profession came into existence. This formulated itself into the hospices set up by the growing Christian Church as it slowly established itself in Europe. This situation continued for several centuries allowing the treatment of disease to continue in the hands of the religious establishments, alchemists or village elders who still possessed the secrets of herbal cures.

Some of the most well known amongst the ancient herbalists of the Western world are Solomon, Dioscorides, who gave us the first Western Materia Medica in the times of Nero, the despotic Roman Emperor, Rucllius, a13th century French translator of Discorides' work, and the 14th century German herbalist, the famous Fuchs (from whom we have the name Fuchsia) as well as another German of the same period Gesner. Herbal medicines were it seems most popular and were in common use well into the 16th and 17th centuries.

This situation continued until the sixteenth century when science began to replace traditional modes of advancement. The Western preoccupation with this new philosophy, which took it further and further away from nature, and in fact set society on a collision course with the same, led it to slowly discard these natural remedies as being obsolete and out-dated. The materialistic approach to life led humankind to adopt a lifestyle contrary to that intended for it. This in turn resulted in the upsurge of newer ailments that found their origins in these changes.

In fact the only field in which modern medical science really progressed was surgery, an area that more ancient forms of medicine had avoided, considering it to be a last resort when all else had failed. This may have been due to religious concerns or just to the fact that it was considered unnatural and relegated it to a lower status much below that of natural healing.

Realising that working against the norms of nature was counterproductive certain more rational physicians began to question this approach to medicine. Most notable amongst them were Dr. Hahnemann, the father of homoeopathy, and Dr. Edward Bach, who also discarded popular medical science to take up more natural forms of healing that included aromatherapy and herbal treatment. Culpeper's English Herbal is evidence enough that prior to the onward march of medical science, the use of common herbs to relive the ailments of mankind had been until that time the most accepted and successful way of dealing with disease and knowledge of these herbs was quite common.

The Greek theories of medicine were based upon ideas developed by the Hippocratic School and further refined by Galen. Their treatment of disease and illness was based upon the theories of the 'four humours'; blood, phlegm, black bile and yellow bile that were qualified by natures and elements.

Natures: —being cold, dry, wet and hot.

Elements: —being water, earth, air and fire.

Blood—was thought to be hot and wet and was related to air

Phlegm—was wet and cold and related to water

Black bile—was cold and dry and related to earth

Yellow bile—was dry and hot and related to fire

Medicines were also categorised according to these same criteria.

Hippocrates theory stated that good health depended upon the humours being in complete balance with each other.

Galen's however stated that there was no such equilibrium and that each person tended towards a particular type of humeral imbalance. This then characterised his temperament, people thus being categorised as being sanguine, phlegmatic, melancholic or choleric. He also felt that the predominance of any one humour could be brought about by external factors like climate, age or lifestyle.

It was believed that the digestion created the humours and that the humour mixture was simply a receptacle for the spirit. There were three spirits: —

The Vital Spirit—in the left ventricle of the heart and by nature hot and dry

The Natural Spirit—located in the liver, hot and wet

The Psyche Spirit—cold and wet located in the brain

Health, according to Galen, consisted in the relative harmony of the humours; illness indicated a disruption of that harmony. Therefore to cure such an illness this balance had to be restored. It was seen that to cure a cold disease hot medicines were given, and to cure a wet disease dry remedies were prescribed.

Medicines were categorised according to the same criteria as the humours; dry and cold; dry and hot; hot and wet; and cold and wet. Since a cold disease indicated for example an excess of black bile, a medicine classified as hot was administered to restore the normal healthy balance.

External factors like climate, food, level of activity, emotional upheaval and others could also influence the humeral balance and physicians always tried to establish a person's circumstances in order to prescribe the correct remedy. This system had a holistic approach and not only the balance of the humours was taken into consideration it also required living in total harmony with one's environment.

The Chinese system also employed the basic concept of treating the body and its ailments in a holistic manner. The ideas and practices of the Chinese System also encompassed the systems that were prevalent in Korea and Japan, though of course there may have been differences in the actual herbs and certain of the techniques used.

The Yellow Emperor (Huang Di) and the Divine Farmer (Shen Nong) are the legendary founders of medicine for the Chinese, though historical sources describing the origin of this system are few. References to Chinese medicine other than the important Mawangdui Texts are to found mainly in philosophical and historical texts such as the Zuozhuan and Zhuangzi. It can therefore be assumed that Chinese Medicine is at best a tradition derived from different and sometimes antithetical sources and not as having a single origin.

Chinese Medicine considers illnesses and cures in the human body as a combination of physical, psychological, emotional, environmental and even cosmic factors. A Taoist physician looks upon illness as caused by a disturbance in a person's relationship with his surroundings, primarily because the person loses quietness (*jing*), which is fundamental to a harmonious life. Thus his primary objective is to use all means at his disposal to restore the person's internal peace and thus achieve a cure.

Chinese Medicine employs a number of techniques for the maintenance of this internal harmony and peace; they include herbal remedies, acupuncture, moxibustion and massage etc. there are eight therapies in all: —

Han—(sweating) making the patient sweat; this method is used when there is a superficial damage, mostly caused by external circumstances

Tu—(vomiting) making the patient vomit; used for instances when the person has been poisoned or when food is not being digested

Xia—(lowering) lowering matter inside the human body by creating downward (outward) movement; used for instances when there is constipation

He—(harmonising) regulating or adjusting one bodily function to the other; for instance when the upper part of the digestive system is not in harmony with the lower part

Wen—(warming) making the temperature in certain parts of the body rise; used when cold is the cause of the disease

Qing—(purifying) clearing heat and purifying the body; applied when heat is the source of illness

Xiao—(dispelling) eliminating or dispersing the causes of disease; used for eliminating blockages on the roads of *qi*, or of other blocked body fluids and material

Bu—(supplying) improving the conditions of *qi*, *xue* (blood fluid) and all functions of the body; accelerating the recovery of someone by giving him more strength

The complex nature of some diseases may require the use of one or more of these therapies in combination to provide a complete cure.

Acupuncture: the practice of inserting needles into various parts of the body to exact a cure.

Moxibustion: the burning of 'moxa' or 'ai' (*Artemisia vulgaris*) directly on the skin, or with an insulation of ginger slices, or in conjunction with acupuncture.

Massage and the use of exercise (qigong): form a vast field of study and demonstrate that the ancient culture of China was extremely developed in its array of curative and preventative methods.

Influenced by the Taoist concept of the bodily functions, the Chinese have come to treat the body as a world within itself. The Taoists also believed that spirits occupied the body's important areas, thus taking care of its different functions. They viewed dreaming as being a temporary separation when the spirit communicates with the celestial spirit world. Taoist rituals and medical practices are concerned with appeasing the '*shen*' or spirit, thus harmonising the body. All medical treatment therefore was aimed at creating harmony between the spirit and the body.

For the Chinese disease means disharmony and the English word 'dis-ease' becomes a perfect translation for the Taoist concept of illness. For the Taoist illness is caused by lack of rest (jing). The *Daodejing* (Tao Te Ching) describes the condition of 'jing' as 'returning to the roots' and 'renewing life'. To achieve this harmony and prevent illness thus the adoption of exercise along with dietary control and the cansideration that a person's life is dependent on his own actions rather than a benevolent God.

To diagnose an illness the Chinese physician adopted four methods; observation of the patient; examination by listening, smelling and tasting; examination by interrogation; and examination by touching, i.e. examination of the pulse, which was given the most importance. The Chinese believe that preserving health and preventing disease is far better than cure. The use of herbal medicines to this end in conjunction with exercise has always been the most preferred in China to prolong life or prevent premature ageing.

Ingredients used in Chinese medicine range from herbs, to minerals and animal components. The nature of these medicines can be cold, hot, warm, or cool (the qi of these medicines). They can also be sour, bitter, sweet, pungent and salty. There are also those which are tasteless and astringent. Each and every taste or nature influence the basic causes of disease (cold, heat etc.) and in a way create a change of condition.

There are also religious therapies adopted by both the Buddhist and Taoist traditions that provide certain mantras which may be uttered by both monks and the laity to promote health and inner comfort.

By far the most sophisticated of all the systems on record, as well as being the best recorded and the most influential of them all, is the Ayurvedic system, which is still very much in use in the Indian sub-continent to the exclusion of western biomedicine. The gift of the Mystical Dhanvantri, worshipped as the celestial fore father of medicine, 'Ayurveda' is composed of two Sanskrit terms, viz., '*ayus*' meaning 'life', and '*veda*' meaning the 'knowledge' and taken together, it means the 'Science of Life'. However in a limited sense, it is always used to imply the 'Science of Medicine'. Charaka has defined Ayurveda as the science through the help of which one can obtain knowledge about the useful and harmful types of life (*hita* and *ahita ayus*), happy and miserable types of life, things which are useful and harmful for such types of life, the span of life as well as the very nature of life. It will be seen from this definition that Ayurveda lays emphasis upon not only leading a life, which is full of happiness, which implies an individualistic attitude but also leading a life, which will be useful to society as a whole. According to ancient Indian texts humankind has a fourfold objective in life: —

1. Dharma (the performance of duties as ordained by the law of nature): these duties are mentioned in various religions as virtuous acts. Thus it appears that sincerely observing the commands of the religion of one's own faith is treated as *sine quo non*-for a happy and healthy life.

2. Artha (accumulation of wealth): to enable one to sustain and fulfill the other objectives, one needs financial support, which has to be acquired by observing legal, moral, and ethical norms.

3. Kama (satisfaction of worldly desires): Ayurveda believes in the existence of past and future lives in addition to the present one. Unfulfilled desires are the source of unhappiness in the present life and thus also in future lives. Therefore it is necessary to that these desires be fulfilled, of course only in accordance with familial, social, cultural and religious prescriptions as well as prohibitions.

4. Moksha (attainment of salvation): when a person becomes free from desire, he attains '*nirvana*' or salvation.

Charaka-samhita summarises this in the form of three *eshanas* (eternal and instinctive desires)—*pranaishana* (desire to have a long and healthy life), *dhanaishana* (desire to acquire wealth), and *paralokaishana* (desire to attain happiness in the next life).

The majority of scholars recognise eight important branches of Ayurveda that include: — ***Kaya-chikitsa*** or Internal Medicine; ***Salya-chikitsa*** or Surgery; ***Salakya-tantra*** or the treatment of diseases of the head and neck; ***Agada-tantra*** or Toxicology; ***Bhuta-vidya*** or the management of seizures by evil spirits and other mental disorders; ***Bala-tantra*** or Paediatrics; ***Rasayana-tantra*** or Geriatrics including Rejuvenation therapy; and ***Vajikarana-tantra*** or the Science of Aphrodisiacs.

There are several other branches that cannot be ignored. Some scholars are of the view that this list should include ***Panchakarma-chikitsa*** (five elimination therapies) as an additional specialised branch and in some medieval works ***Dravya-guna*** (Materia-medica) is also described as one of the specialised branches. In the Jivaka's ***Amrita-hridaya-astanga-guhyopadesha***, ***Matri-roga-chikitsa*** (the treatment of maternal diseases) is described as one of these specialised branches too.

Ayurvedic therapeutics recognises only the use of natural ingredients. These include herbs, metals and animal products. Plants that are grown in their natural surroundings are the most preferred, though due to supply and demand differences some of the most used herbs may be cultivated commercially and it must be understood that this will only be under the most natural conditions without the use of chemical fertilizers or insecticides. It may therefore be stated that the use of synthetic chemicals is categorically prohibited in Ayurveda. It has been found that these natural products are relatively more homologous to the tissue elements of the body and are more easily digested, absorbed and readily assimilated by the tissues to produce their therapeutic effects. There are also naturally produced substitutes that can be used in the case of non-availability of any of the prescribed herbs.

Although synthetic and unnatural remedies may at times help people to overcome pain or other such ailments more quickly, in the long run they tend to damage the vital organs of the body. Natural cures and products used in Ayurveda do not have these damaging side effects. Rather because of their homologous nature they help to tone up those organs.

Diagnostics in Ayurveda comprises mainly identifying the ailments simply by examining the pulse and urine samples. It certainly does not require the lengthy and expensive procedures that are adopted by the modern Western physicians before they arrive at any prognosis. It is unfortunate that we have all come to accept these expensive and sometimes lengthy procedures as being part and parcel of our treatment. Also this has become an excuse for the more commercially minded doctors to over prescribe and sometimes recommend unnecessary medicines that we could well do without.

The Ayurvedic approach to health care in itself is completely opposed to the more modern systems of medicine. Its basic approach is to provide an environment within the body itself that will keep it free from disease, whereas most Western systems work on the premise that they have to treat illnesses as they occur. Therefore their working style becomes more a symptomatic approach rather than a search for basic causes. The interest in Ayurvedic medicines has of course increased a great deal as researchers search for more natural medicines that do not have the more serious side effects that have been experienced with the highly potent chemical based drugs, which have become so prolific these days. The holistic reasoning that Ayurvedic practitioners have adopted reflects their understanding that each individual is a complete replica of the universe as a whole and any form of treatment has to take in to consideration many more factors than most systems of medicine do. Ayurveda is therefore, in the modern sense, more eco-friendly and less harmful, thus providing a more natural and acceptable system that not only provides us with natural medicines but also takes into account the overall physical and mental condition of the patient.

Ginger, like many other medicinal herbs, is one of those common and garden kitchen condiments that all of us tend to overlook. Used liberally in most South Asian dishes it adds spice and flavour to the vast gamut of the curried food available there. Ginger is one of those common and seemingly insignificant root tubers that can almost grow wild in your back yard. It goes well with honey dew melons when its dried powder is sprinkled over the succulent slices served before the main course meals. Candied ginger is also used in confectionery and if simply chewed gives one suffering from a niggling cough immediate though temporary relief.

Common names: Black ginger, race ginger, African ginger. Parts used: Root.

Medicinal properties: Stimulant, pungent, carminative, aromatic, sialagogue, condiment and diaphoretic.

Description and uses: When taken hot, ginger is excellent in cases of suppressed menstruation. Chewing a little of the root stimulates the salivary glands and is very useful in paralysis of the tongue and is also good for sore throats. Prevents griping and is good for diarrhoea, colds, la grippe, chronic bronchitis, coughs, dyspepsia, gas and fermentation, cholera, gout and nausea when combined with stronger laxative herbs. Produces perspiration when taken hot.

It should be noted that in Ayurveda there is a definite distinction made between fresh ginger root and its dried form (sonth). To make this clear we will refer to this form as dried ginger, or dry ginger, to allow our readers to be able to easily identify the two forms.

GINGER; ZINGIBER OFFICINALIS ROSC.

(Zingiberaceae) Rhizomous herb

Chukku, Inchi
The hot root
Ginger
Employed as a hot remedy for coughs, asthma, worms, leprosy and other skin diseases. Almost all of the Ayurvedic medicines has ginger as an ingredient. Very effective in stomach complaints.

Sanskrit—Ardraka; Hindi—Adrak, Sounth

Ginger has been a renowned root for more than two thousand years. When you make it as a tea, it warms you from head to toe.

Also called 'Vishvaushadha' in Sanskrit, ginger is anti-rheumatic, stimulant, digestive, laxative, good for eyes and throat and nutritive. Its purgative properties destroy intestinal worms, which are then expelled through faeces. Ginger is a good tonic for the intestines. Compared to other poisonous drugs, ginger juice is safe and free from ill effects.

Beneficent Part: Root.

Properties: Alkaloids, Mucilage, Phenols and Volatile Oil.

Medicinal Values: Antispasmodic, Antiseptic, Carminative, Circulatory Stimulant, Expectorant and Tonic.

Analysis of Contents

Water	80.9%
Protein	2.3%
Fat	0.9%
Carbohydrates	12.3%
Iron	2.6mg/100gm

In addition to the above nutrients ginger contains vitamin 'A' and Vitamin 'C', and phosphorous etc., in small quantities.

Use: Three or four teaspoonfuls of ginger juice mixed with a very small quantity of mineral salt and a few drops of lemon juice taken half an hour before meals works as an excellent appetiser.

Ginger juice stimulates the secretion of digestive juices. This helps digestion and prevents gas troubles.

Benefits: Juice or small pieces of ginger taken before meals eliminate gas. It dislodges coughs and exterminates catarrh and cold. It corrects cardiac disorders and allays all abdominal disorders. Ginger juice is also helpful in oedema, uric troubles, jaundice, piles, asthma, cough, dropsy and a whole host of other diseases. In the opinion of a number of Ayurvedic experts, a regular intake of ginger can prove very beneficial in preventing malignancy. Some have even claimed success in their treatment of cancer by the introduction of ginger into the regimen of medicines prescribed. Ginger also gives relief in catarrh and sinus problems.

Used as a Tea

Arthritis, Rheumatism Gout and Osteoporosis: Ginger warms and comforts the body and increases the blood flow to cleanse toxins and promote healing. It has a good reputation as a remedy for arthritis, rheumatism, gout and osteoporosis.

Cold and Chills, Cold hands and Feet: Ginger is a warming tea that is also a mild expectorant, which is very beneficial for cold conditions that include colds, chills and congestion. It's a fine tea to take when you feel cold, lack an appetite, or have cold hands or feet.

Heart Health: Ginger is a gem for the heart. It lowers cholesterol, stabilises blood pressure and heart functions, helps to prevent clotting, and reduces the risk of heart attacks and strokes.

Nausea and Motion Sickness: Ginger stops nausea and queasiness better than any pill. A cup of ginger tea before you travel will calm you all over.

The homoeopathic Materia Medica tells us that Zingiber is suited to states of debility in the digestive tract like diarhoea, dysentry, food poisoning, hepatitis as well as asthma.

Weight Control and Digestion: Ginger stimulates saliva, digestive enzymes for proteins and fats, and it increases metabolic heat to burn calories.

Uses Through the Ages: In the eighteenth century, ginger was used in blends to balance other herbs and soothe the stomach. In China it is used for colds and chills, and it's considered a "yang" tonic for spleen energy. In India too it is a very common remedy for coughs and colds and Ayurveda has spoken highly of it used especially in its dried form.

Harmony Tea: A marvellous way to reap the benefits of ginger and moderate its heat is in a blend with peppermint. That way the warming effect of ginger is tamed by the cooling effect of peppermint, for an exhilarating brew that also brings harmony.

Used as a Bath

Ginger Bath: Made from freshly grated ginger roots, this bath stimulates circulation, alleviates aches and pains, breaks a cold, helps arthritis and warms the body. A ginger bath is also wonderful for influenzas, gout, bursitis, feeling cold and tiredness. Immerse the whole body in a tub full of hot water, $^1/_3$ of it being ginger tea.

The same bath may be made in smaller quantities and used as a soak for aching, sore, swollen or numb hands, feet or any other body part. A hot ginger footbath eases sore and aching feet, stimulates the circulation and warms the body and helps energy and mental tiredness.

The ginger footbath is also useful in causing sweating to break fevers and colds. To do this, sit in a chair with the feet in a tub of ginger tea. Then wrap blankets about the head and body, encompassing the tub of ginger tea. Leave in place for 5-10 minutes after a sweat has occurred. Then rinse off, dress in clean clothes and go to bed well covered.

Radish Leaves Bath: A hipbath in radish leaf water is specific for bladder infections, acute or chronic. It is good for any other genito-reproductive disorders such as endometritis, leucorrhoea and menstrual difficulties. In the hipbath, only the pelvis or hips are immersed in the tub with the feet and upper area covered and hanging out of the tub. Daikon radish leaves are best to use since they are more stimulating than most radishes, but any radish leaves may be used.

Chop up a large handful of radish leaves, add 1 tablespoon of freshly grated ginger and tie up in a thin cloth bag. Put under the faucet (tap) or simply pour hot water over them to fill the tub. Soak the hips for 20 to 30 minutes.

Ginger Fomentation: Ginger fomentation is excellent for congestion, sprains, cramps, pains, coldness, swellings, colds, influenzas, coughs, excessive mucus and strained muscles. It is also very effective for drawing out blood toxins and stimulating the circulation. Ginger is a very warming herb, which also moves blood, energy, fluids and toxins.

Place over lower abdomen and perineum during childbirth to help prevent tearing and stop pain; place over the chest for congested lungs, cough, asthma and pneumonia; over the abdomen for pains, spasms, poor digestion, coldness, bladder infections (in a cold person) and menstrual cramps; over the lower back for pain and ache, lowered immunity and energy and poor digestion; over any other part of the body where there is congestion, sprain, cramps or pain.

Used as a massage Oil

Ginger Sesame Oil: This oil activates the functions of the blood capillaries, circulation and nerve reactions. Use for aches and pains, headaches or pain in the spine or joints by massaging it into the skin. It can also be used for earaches by placing 2-3 drops of the oil on cotton wool, which is then placed in the aching ear for several hours keeping the head tipped sideways for a while until the oil has penetrated. Leave the cotton wool and oil in the ear for a few hours

It is also useful for scalp diseases and dandruff. Rub ginger sesame oil on the scalp and leave it there for at least 8 hours or overnight. Then wash with a herbal shampoo. Do this 2-3 times a week.

To make, use a mixture of equal amounts of sesame oil and fresh ginger juice. To extract the ginger juice, grate the ginger and express the juice by squeezing it through a cheesecloth.

Used in Combination

Trikatu: Trikatu is a traditional Ayurvedic (East Indian) formula composed of three spices: (dry) ginger, black pepper and pippili (Indian long pepper). Anise seeds may be used in place of pippili where it is not available. Equal parts of the powders are combined and taken with warm milk, or mixed with enough honey to form a paste, and then eaten.

Spicy and stimulating, Trikatu is useful to stimulate the body's energy and circulation and to dry wet conditions. It helps dry mucus and so is fabulous for colds, influenzas, mucous congestion, lung ailments, sore throat, allergies and cough, all derived from coldness. It helps reduce fat, aids digestion and circulation and warms internally. A specific remedy for clear damp, discharges that often occur in cold, damp-climates, Trikatu should be taken in winter by nearly everyone living in such environments and then suspended during the warm summer months.

Ginger Milk: It is a tasty treat, which is also very warming to the body. It is made by first scalding a cup of milk and adding a ½ teaspoon of honey and a ½ teaspoon of powdered ginger, the mucous producing and congesting properties of milk are negated, and the body receives a warming nutritive tonic instead.

Ginger Tea: Ginger tea is useful for indigestion, gas, influenzas, colds, sore throats, poor circulation, coughs, lung-congestion, low energy and lack of appetite. If used at the first sign of any of these ailments it will generally knock them out of the system. After a condition has developed or ripened the tea should be ingested several times a day until the problem goes away. To make ginger tea grate two inches of fresh ginger root and make it into an infusion with one pint of water.

Ginger may also be added to your daily cup of tea or along with various other herbs to produce a delicious and spicy tea that is traditionally enjoyed in India. Because it is spicy and stimulating it is good for poor circulation, coldness, low or poor appetite, poor digestion, gas, bloatedness and colds. It is also a wonderful winter beverage as a preventative to these conditions. There are people who make a big pot of it and use it as their main winter tea daily. For those with heat signs of any sort, it may be too spicy and should therefore be avoided.

To make it simply combine freshly grated ginger, seven pepper corns, one cinnamon stick, five cloves, fifteen cardamom seeds and the peel of one orange with one pint of water. Cover the pot and simmer for ten minutes. Add a half a cup of milk and simmer covered another ten minutes. Strain and sweeten with honey. It is usually made in India using black tea. However for those who wish to avoid the caffeine intake, you may make it with herbs alone.

Scallion-Ginger Tea: for the common cold, make a tea using the white part of two scallions (spring onions) and one teaspoon of freshly grated ginger root to one cup of water. Drink freely as needed.

Asthma: Elecampane root tea is effective, to which can be added ½ part each of ginger and liquorice, 1-2 teaspoons of herbs to each cup of boiling water; or equal parts of thyme and comfrey root can be used in a similar fashion. For severe asthmatic attacks, always consult a medical practitioner.

For relief from asthma attacks prepare a decoction of five grams of the inflorescences of the Tulasi and ten grams of dry ginger in water, allow it to cool and add some honey. Take two or three times as necessary.

Backache: Apply ginger paste and then eucalyptus oil to the affected area.

Boils: To bring a skin boil to a head, apply cooked onions as a poultice or apply a paste of ginger powder and turmeric (½ a teaspoon of each) directly to the boil.

Bronchitis: Take warm water with ginger, honey and lemon juice in the morning, or take warm water with garlic and onion juices. Besides take radish, cabbage, beetroot, cucumber and carrot juices. Of course you should avoid smoking at all costs.

Cancer: Opinions are divided as to which juices give the maximum benefit in cases of cancer. Normally these juices are beneficial— the juices of carrot, grape, beetroot, apple, ginger, papaya, and tomato. One should try to maintain the health of the liver. Magnet therapy is also recommended.

Cold: Lemonated warm water should be taken. The juices of ginger, orange, carrot, radish and garlic etc., can also be taken. Water vapour is also very useful.

Common colds: Severe—Take 1 tablespoon of grated fresh ginger with 1 teaspoon of cinnamon and teaspoon of liquorice and boil in one quart of water for ten minutes. Take one cup every three hours sweetened with a little honey.

Whatever the reasons for the cold, Tulasi will help you to get rid of it and its concomitant fever within a few days. To do this you must prepare a hot decoction of dry ginger, black pepper, Tulasi leaves and jaggery. This decoction should be taken every two to three hours.

If you are suffering with a chronic cold, drink a hot decoction of cloves, cinnamon, dry ginger, black pepper, Tulasi and cardamom every morning and evening.

If the cold has been caused by a drenching in the rain, or excessive humidity in the air, drinking a decoction of Tulasi, dry ginger, cloves, cinnamon and black pepper three or four times in a day will effect a cure.

A mixture of fifteen grams of Tulasi juice, twenty-five grams of pure honey and five grams of ginger juice taken in doses of twenty-five to sixty drops, will cure coughs and fevers.

Licking a paste obtained by crushing equal quantities of Tulasi inflorescences and ginger and mixing them with honey relieves a dry cough. This should be done three or five times a day.

A paste formed by grinding Tulasi seeds, onions and ginger and mixing it with honey is beneficial in dry coughs and infantile asthma. The paste is to be licked.

If phlegm has become too viscid and coughing cannot bring it up for expectoration, lick a paste formed by mixing the juices of Tulasi, onions and ginger with an equal quantity of honey. This will encourage the expectoration of the phlegm and thus clear the respiratory channels.

Boil eleven Tulasi leaves, two or three black pepper corns, a small piece of ginger and a pinch of rock salt in a cupful of water till only half a cup is left. Take the extract off the fire and strain it. Drinking this in three portions will cure coughs and colds.

Constipation: Severe—Take an infusion of rhubarb root (1.teaspoon per cup) along with ¼ teaspoon each of ginger and liquorice (increase dosage if necessary). Moderate—Take 1-2 teaspoons of Psyllum husk powder in a cup of warm water before sleep. Mild—Take 1teaspoon of Ghee in a cup of warm milk.

Cough: Drink elecampane root tea, to which smaller amounts of ginger and liquorice can be added, 1-2 teaspoons of the herb to each cup of boiling water; sweeten with honey. For mucus, prepare a tea of ½ a teaspoon of ginger powder, cloves and cinnamon, per cup; sweeten with honey.

Diarrhoea: Blend together ½ cup of yogurt and ½ cup of water to which 1-teaspoon of grated fresh ginger has been added and a little nutmeg. For dysentery, take equal parts of barberry and raspberry leaves along with a ½ part of nutmeg. Make an infusion of 2-3 teaspoons per cup and take every few hours until condition improves.

Gas (abdominal): Make an infusion of cardamom, fennel and ginger in equal parts, 1 teaspoon per cup, to which a pinch of asafoetida may be added.

Haemorrhoids: Drink ½ a teaspoon of aloe vera gel with a little ginger twice a day until the Haemorrhoids disappear.

Headaches: For general relief from headaches, a paste of ginger powder, mixed with water and heated, is applied to the forehead. A burning sensation may possibly occur but it will not be harmful.

The following may be used for relief of specific types of headaches. Sinus headaches related to kapha can be relieved by applying a ginger paste to the forehead sinuses. Temporal headaches indicate an excess of pitta in the stomach. They can be relieved by drinking a tea of cumin and coriander seeds, ½ a teaspoon of each, in one cup of hot water. At the same time apply sandalwood oil or sandalwood paste to the temples. Occipital headaches indicate toxins in the colon. Take 2 teaspoons of flaxseed before sleep in one cup of warm milk. At the same time apply ginger paste behind the ears (mastoid process).

Take ginger juice; also the juices of carrots, beetroot cucumber, tomato, cabbage and apple may be taken to great effect.

Indigestion: Lemon juice in warm water should be taken on an empty stomach in the morning. Take a teaspoonful of ginger half an hour before meals. The juices of pineapple, papaya, cucumber and cabbage should also be taken on a regular basis. A blend of carrot, beetroot and spinach juices is also indicated.

Take 2-3 "00" capsules of Trikatu (equal parts of black pepper, Indian long pepper or as a substitute cayenne, and ginger powder) with a little warm water before meals. This is for loss or lack of appetite, poor assimilation and malabsorption. For hyperacidity take 2-3 "00" capsules of equal parts of gentian, barberry, and liquorice after meals.

Loss of appetite: Lemon water should be taken in the morning. In addition to this bitter gourd, carrot and ginger juices can also be taken. Constipation should be relieved and plenty of physical exercise should be undertaken.

Migraine: Take a glassful of water mixed with lemon and ginger juice. Perform Shakasana for 15 minutes every day without fail.

Muscle strain (upper body): An enema of 1 cup calamus oil may be injected into the rectum. Retain for 30 minutes. For general muscle strain apply warm ginger paste with turmeric (one teaspoon of ginger with ½ teaspoon of turmeric) to the affected area twice a day.

Pain external: Apply a ginger compress. To prepare a ginger compress, combine 2 teaspoons of ginger powder with 1 teaspoon of turmeric powder and add enough water to make a paste. Warm the paste and spread it evenly on a piece of gauze or cotton cloth. Then place the cloth on the affected area and apply a bandage over it. Keep it on overnight.

Pneumonia: Take immediate medical treatment. Take warm water with ginger, lemon and honey or as an alternative take warm water with garlic and onion juices. The juices of basil, mosambi, orange and carrot are also recommended.

Sinus congestion: Inhale a pinch of calamus root powder or apply ginger paste to the affected area. One can also inhale the steam from a tea of ginger or eucalyptus leaves. A few drops of ginger juice poured into the nose give sure relief to headaches.

Throat troubles: Take warm water with honey and lemon juice in the morning. Also you can take pineapple but allow the movement of the juice in your mouth before swallowing it. At the same time you may take a mixture of carrot, beetroot and cucumber juice. Take a glassful of warm water with a spoonful each of garlic, ginger and onion juices or an infusion of the same. A spoonful of green turmeric juice is also very useful.

Toothache will be relieved if a piece of ginger is rubbed on the ailing tooth.

Sleep (excess): In the evening drink an infusion of ½ teaspoon of calamus root powder and ¼ teaspoon of ginger powder per cup of water; or, alternatively, drink a cup of basil leaf tea.

Sprain: Massage with equal amounts of garlic and almond oil. In a hot bath, add ½ a cup of ginger powder and ½ cup of baking soda. To this add 1 teaspoon of eucalyptus oil. Sit for 15 minutes.

Apply warm ginger paste with turmeric (1 teaspoon of ginger with ½ teaspoon of turmeric) to the affected area twice a day.

If there are dark spots on your face add some lemon juice to Tulasi juice and apply the mixture to your face. Allow it to dry and then wash it off with clear water. If this is done regularly every morning and evening, the spots will disappear and your face will become clean fresh and glowing. An equal amount of ginger juice can be substituted for the lemon juice.

In cases of dry cough the patient should lick up a paste of Tulasi shoots, ginger and honey. It should not be washed down with water.

If the child complains of abdominal pains a slightly warmed mixture of Tulasi and ginger juice will provide relief.

Five grams each of Tulasi juice, ajwain (king's cumin, thymol) and turmeric are ground to a very fine paste and added to twenty-five grams of honey. The mixture is then stored in a glass jar. Thirty to sixty drops of this mixture administered two to three times a day to a child suffering with cough and cold will bring a great deal of relief.

In cases of the distention of the stomach due to the excessive formation of gas administer five to ten grams of Tulasi juice (according to age) to give relief.

In cases of colic, dry ginger powder mixed with Tulasi juice will bring relief.

Influenza and coughs can be cured by administering thirty to sixty drops of a mixture composing of Tulasi juice, ajwain (king's cumin, thymol) ginger juice and honey.

The juices of Tulasi and ginger warmed together and administered with honey when cold will keep children healthy and prevent retention of urine and stool, constipation, indigestion, vomiting, hiccoughs, shortness of breath, coughs, fevers and colds etc.

Repeated administration of a mixture of Tulasi, onion and garlic juices all over the body is an excellent remedy for inflammation caused by wind.

A patient suffering with tetanus should be made to drink a mixture of the juices of garlic, ginger, onions and Tulasi leaves. This mixture should be applied all over the body too. This treatment will cure tetanus.

Taking ten grams of Tulasi juice thrice daily, morning, noon and evening can cure malaria. Alternatively ten grams of Tulasi juice mixed with five grams of ginger juice can work equally as well.

The juices of Tulasi and ginger mixed with honey will always help to stimulate the appetite and help to cure colds, fevers and pneumonia as well.

Considerable benefit can be obtained by taking ten grams of a mixture of the equal parts of powdered Tulasi leaves, ajwain (king's cumin-thymol) and dry ginger with some honey three times a day.

Boil five Tulasi leaves with five black pepper corns and five grams of ginger in a cupful of water. Add sugar to taste and drink whilst it is still hot. Do this every morning and evening for quick relief.

Grind eleven Tulasi leaves, nine black pepper corns, thirty grams of ajwain (king's cumin—thymol), and fifty grams of dry ginger in a mortar. Heat up a clay pot and pour in the above mixture and expose your body to the vapours that are given off. When the temperature comes down to a tolerable level add a little rock salt to the mixture and drink it down. This will cure almost any fever.

Those who are subject to relapses of malarial fevers preceded by cold rigours should take a decoction prepared from five grams each of Tulasi, mint and ginger.

CONCLUSION

To adapt one's life to the environment around has been man's greatest attribute. Unfortunately whilst doing so he has forgotten many of the benefits of keeping his life especially his eating habits, as simple as possible. All societies have their festivals and religious days that allow one to enjoy ones food a little more by enjoying exotic dishes and special treats. This is good, for as they say change is as good as a holiday, but as you cannot live a lifetime of holidays so if you want to remain healthy you cannot abuse your system either. A certain amount of temperance with regards to eating habits has to be observed to guarantee reasonable health. But so it is true of all aspects of life.

The use of such common and garden herbs like ginger may in many ways simplify your life as well as removing the burden of extended doctor's bills from your pocket. Not only does ginger enhance your food but if used properly it can also provide you with a cheap and readily available source of medicine for a vast variety of illnesses. The conscious use of such herbs will benefit you and very rarely harm your delicate constitution. Obviously there are certain conditions that will negate the use of ginger and one should always consult practicing herbalists whenever in doubt.

THERAPEUTIC PROCEDURES

How To Make Plasters

A plaster is a herbal mash that is wrapped up in a protective cloth or combined in a thick base material, such as oil or Vaseline, and then placed on the skin. It is first placed in the cloth or oil because the herbs used in a plaster are stronger and might burn or extremely irritate the skin if they were put directly on it. Mustard and garlic are two common examples.

Plasters are good for muscular spasms, swellings, arthritis, rheumatism, tumours, fevers, mucous congestion in the chest, bronchitis and pneumonia. They can be used in treating enlarged glands and organs (neck, breast, groin, kidney, liver and prostrate) and various eruptions (boils and abscesses).

Baths: How to Prepare

Method 1—yields a stronger bath:

1. Chop up or grate desired herbs
2. Make an infusion or decoction, as appropriate
3. Add the tea to the hot bath
4. Soak and enjoy

Method 2—yields a weaker bath

1. Chop up or grate desired herbs
2. Place in a thin cloth bag
3. Tie bag under faucet (tap) or simply pour your hot water over it whilst filling the tub or just place the bag directly in the tub.

If using method one then prepare two gallons (approximately 10 litres) of herb tea. If using method two use two to six ounces (grams) of herbs, depending on the strength desired and herbs used. Weaker herbs need larger quantities while stimulating herbs can be used more sparingly.

Take baths as needed.

Bath herbs are not stored after use. A bath may be made from any herbs left on hand and is an especially good use for herbs stored a long time when their medicinal values and actions have weakened, usually within a year or two (depending on the form in which they are stored).

How To Prepare Tea

Tea is a very broad term to describe a preparation of herbs to be ingested. It is a very popular way of imbibing the health giving qualities that herbs offer. It is also a method well tried and recommended by the most ancient of medical systems. The Chinese, Japanese, Tibetan, and Korean systems (where tea drinking socially is a part of their culture) as well as the Indian systems all recommend preparations of herbs that come under the heading of teas. Even in Europe, tea preparations have been recorded and there are many references to different kinds of floral and herbal teas that are served not only as healers but also as tonics to the debilitated to encourage swift recoveries.

A) INFUSIONS

1. Bring water to boil and then turn off the heat
2. In the meantime put your herbs in a teapot or container
3. Pour the boiled water over the herbs in the teapot
4. Put a tight lid on the container to prevent the volatile oils from escaping and put in a warm place
5. Let the mixture sit (steep) for fifteen minutes
6. Strain tea by pouring the liquid through a strainer into a cup and drink

B) DECOCTIONS

1. Place herbs directly in water and stir well
2. Bring the water to a boil, then turn the heat down to simmer
3. Simmer the herbs for 30-60 minutes (30 minutes for coarse leaves and up to 60 minutes for stems, roots and barks). Usually the water will decrease by half due to evaporation
4. Strain tea by pouring the herb water through a strainer into a cup and drink

C) SUN TEA

Preparation:

1. Wash the leaves or flowers well and place them in a clear glass jar
2. Fill the jar to the top with water and then screw the lid on to the jar tightly
3. Place the jar in the sun for four or more hours as desired
4. Strain and drink

Quantities:

Use one cup of your herb mixture or the equivalent of about twelve tea bags for a one-gallon (approximately four and a half litre) jar. For a medicinal tea, use one ounce (approximately 28.5 grams) to one pint (approximately half a litre) of water. For a strong tea, leave the jar in the sun for the entire day; for weak tea, just leave it for four hours.

Dosage:

Drink three cups a day or as desired for beverage.

Storage:

Store refrigerated for up to three days.

HOW TO PREPARE FOMENTATIONS

1. Make tea out of herbs, either infusion or decoction
2. Dip a small cloth, (such as a washcloth) into the tea and allow it to soak for five to ten minutes to absorb the herbal tea
3. Using a pair of tongs, lift cloth out of tea. Quickly wring out and put over the part of the body where fomentation is desired
4. Immediately cover the cloth with a towel. Place a hot water bottle or heating pad over the towel and cover everything with another towel so that all is kept warm
5. Leave the fomentation in place for at least twenty minutes. If using castor oil and you plan to leave the fomentation on overnight, then protect the bed with several towels or a plastic covering before lying down

Quantity:

Make about two to four cups of tea for the fomentation, using two to four ounces of herbs respectively, depending on body area covered and number of fomentations to be done.

Dosage:

You may want to put a fomentation on more than once. Fomentations can be left on for twenty minutes or more: then another cloth soaking in tea can be placed over the same area. Leave the second compress on for another twenty minutes. Fomentations can be applied as needed. Be sure to keep them warm.

Storage:

Fomentations are not stored but made when needed.

HOW TO PREPARE MILK DECOCTIONS

Method one—simple and quick form

1. Powder desired herbs.
2. Add the herbs to milk in a pan, stirring well.
3. Slowly heat milk and simmer for five to ten minutes over low heat.
4. Strain large herb parts if desired. Cool and drink as it is.

Method two—traditionally used in Ayurvedic medicine

1. Combine one ounce (28.5 grams) of whole herbs with one cup of milk and four cups of water in a pan.
2. Bring to the boil and cook slowly over a low flame until all the water has evaporated.
3. Strain and cool.

Quantities:

Use one teaspoon of herbs to one cup of milk in method one.

Dosage:

Drink one cup of medicated milk two to three times a day.

Storage:

Milk will last one or two days refrigerated.

HOW TO PREPARE HERBAL OILS

Method one:

1. Rub fresh or dried herbs between palms of hands to break down herbs (called "bruising" herbs).
2. Place herbs in a glass jar.
3. Pour chosen oil(s) over herbs. Cover jar with a tight lid.
4. Shake the jar so that herbs and oil(s) mix together. Do this for at least two weeks.
5. After two weeks, strain the oil(s) by covering a kitchen colander with a piece of cheesecloth. Place the colander in a big bowl. Pour herbal oil into the colander. The herbs will collect in the cheesecloth while the oil will run through into the bowl. If there are still herbs in the oil then repeat the procedure. Squeeze the herbs in the cheesecloth

to release any oil remaining and extract the maximum amount of oil.

6. Pour the contents of the bowl into a clean glass jar and cover tightly. Now you have a herbal oil ready to use.
7. To preserve add tincture of benzoin or vitamin E

Method two:

1. Same as step one above.
2. Place bruised herbs in oil in a pan. Slowly heat and cook the herbs gently until crispy, about a half to one hour.
3. Strain the oil(s) by covering a kitchen colander with a piece of cheesecloth. Place the colander in a big bowl. Pour herbal oil into the colander. The herbs will collect in the cheesecloth while the oil will run through into the bowl. If there are still herbs in the oil then repeat the procedure. Squeeze the herbs in the cheesecloth to release any oil remaining and extract the maximum amount of oil.
4. Pour the contents of the bowl into a clean glass jar and cover tightly. Now you have a herbal oil ready to use.

5. To preserve add tincture of benzoin or vitamin E

Method three—lengthier, but yields a superior oil:

The proportion of herbs to oil is different, and water is added to extract additional medicinal properties into the oil. This is an Ayurvedic method of making herbal oils.

1. Same as step one above.
2. Place one part of herbs to four of oil and sixteen parts of water in a pan.
3. Shake the jar so that herbs and oil(s) mix together. Do this for at least two weeks.
4. After two weeks, strain the oil(s) by covering a kitchen colander with a piece of cheesecloth. Place the colander in a big bowl. Pour herbal oil into the colander. The herbs will collect in the cheesecloth while the oil will run through into the bowl. If there are still herbs in the oil then repeat the procedure. Squeeze the herbs in the cheesecloth to release any oil remaining and extract the maximum amount of oil.

5. Pour the contents of the bowl into a clean glass jar and cover tightly. Now you have a herbal oil ready to use.
6. To preserve add tincture of benzoin or vitamin E.

Quantities:
Use four ounces of dried herbs or eight ounces of fresh herbs to each pint of oil. Add a quarter of a teaspoonful of benzoin to each cup of oil or 400 IU of vitamin E per cup of oil as a preservative.

Dosage:
Oils do not have a dosage limit since they are used on the body. Overuse, however, can be messy and stain clothes or furniture.

Storage:
Oils will last about one year. Store in glass jars in a cool and dark place.

Another easier method though a little time consuming.

First, select the herbs that you wish to add in your oil. Make a decoction of the same. Strain off the liquid and pour into a pan with the same amount of oil. Slowly heat the mixture of oil and the herbal decoction until all the water has evaporated.

The oil may now be stored in a coloured glass bottle for further use.

The ratio of the herbs to be used in the decoction should be about a half an ounce of herbs to one cup of water.

HOW TO PREPARE A HERBAL POULTICE

1. Choose the herb(s) to be used and powder them.
2. Add a little bit of hot water, herbal tea, liniment or a tincture to the powdered herbs and mix to form a thick paste. If all the herbs are not powdered, make them into a tea first and add some to the rest of the powdered herbs.
3. Apply the paste to the skin. Cover right away with gauze bandage and tie or tape in place. Or you may apply the paste to the gauze bandage first and then apply to the skin area. Leave there for several hours or overnight. If needed, replace with another poultice until the problem is healed or removed. Keep arm with hot water bottle or heating pad.

Quantity:
This depends largely on the area to be covered, and if fresh or powdered herbs are to be used. For example an area approximately four square inches will require half an ounce of powdered herb(s) and two tablespoons of liquid.

Dosage:
Some poultices need to be reapplied and kept on for several days. Usually however, they are applied from twenty minutes to several hours or overnight.

Storage:
Poultices are made as needed and never stored.

Some Factors That Weaken the Body And Predispose It To Illness

- Refined foods, such as white flour, white sugar, white rice, white pasta, refined salt
- Chemicals and preservatives in foods
- Extensive use of canned foods
- Frequent indulgence in "junk foods"
- Polluted air and water
- Proximity to major electrical wiring anywhere in the home, or living close to power plants

- Excessive noise
- Stress-causing situations or conditions
- Job-stress or incompatibility
- Relationship problems
- Proximity to colour T.V. or computer monitors
- Extensive computer use without screening of the monitors
- Living near toxic waste dumps
- Frequent use of antibiotics
- Synthetic fibres in clothing and home and office furnishings
- Fast-paced life
- Carcinogenic pollutants from material built in the home or office
- Side effects of drugs
- Mercury amalgam fillings in teeth

Self-Inquiry Questions

Do I truly want to get better?
Am I ready to be healed, to be different than I am now?
And am I willing to do the things necessary to make these changes?
Do I try to sabotage my healing process? If so why?

Why do I continue my harmful habits? What do they give me that I don't get otherwise?

Do I have enough love in my life?

Do I get enough attention in my life?

Am I satisfied emotionally, spiritually, physically, creatively or mentally?

How important am I to me?

Do I feel good about myself, and my life?

Do I allow the world to control and dominate me? Or am I involved in my healing?

What unresolved issues am I carrying around from my childhood or any other time of my life?

Do I like my work or my job?

Am I happy with my career?

Are my relationships satisfying?

What is my true heart's desire?

What changes can I make to start bringing more satisfaction into my life in the areas that are lacking?

What can I do to assure that I follow the changes necessary for improving my health?

What specific help can I seek to make these changes?

Desirable weights for men and women of 25 and over

Weight in pounds (in indoor clothing), Height in feet and inches and approximate metric equivalents in brackets.

Height '(in shoes)	Small-frame	Medium-frame	Large-frame
Men			
5' 2" (158.5cm)	112-120 (50.7-54.4kg)	118-129 (53.5-58.5kg)	126-141(57.1-63.9kg)
3" (160cm)	115-123 (52.1-55kg)	121-133 (54.5-60kg)	129-144 (58.5-65.3kg)
4" (162.6cm)	118-126 (53.5-57.1kg)	124-136 (56.2-61.6kg)	132-148 (59.8-67.1kg)
5" (165cm)	121-129 (54.5-58.5kg)	127-139 (57.5-63kg)	135-152 (61.2-68.9kg)
6" (167.6cm)	124-133 (56.2-60kg)	130-143 (58.9-64.8kg)	138-156 (62.5-70.7kg)
7" (170cm)	128-137 (58-62.1kg)	134-147 (60.7-66.7kg)	142-156 (64.3-70.7kg)
8" (172.7cm)	132-141 (50-54kg)	138-152(62.5-68.9kg)	147-166 (60.7-75.2kg)
9" (175cm)	136-145 (61.2-65.7kg)	142-156(64.3-70.7kg)	151-170 (68.4-77kg)
10" (177.8cm)	140-150 (63.4-68kg)	146-160(66.2-72.5kg)	155-174(70.2-78.9kg)
11" (180cm)	144-154 (65.3-69.8kg)	150-165(68-74.8kg)	159-179(72.1-81.1kg)
6' 0" (182.8cm)	148-158 (67.1-71.6kg)	154-170(69.8-77kg)	164-184(74.3-83.4kg)
1" (185.4cm)	152-162 (68.9-73.4kg)	158-175(71.6-79.3kg)	168-189(76.1-85.7kg)
2" (188cm)	156-167 (70.7-75.7kg)	162-180(73.4-81.6kg)	173-194(78.4-87.9kg)
3" (190.5cm)	160-171 (72.5-77.5kg)	167-185(75.7-83.9kg)	178-199(80.7-90.2kg)
4" (193cm)	164-175 (74.3-79.3kg)	172-190(78-86.1kg)	182-204(82.5-92.5kg)
Women			
4'10" (147cm)	92-98 (41.7-44.4kg)	96-107 (43.5-48.5kg)	104-119 (47-53.9kg)
11" (149.8cm)	94-101 (42.6-45.8kg)	98-110 (44.4-49.8kg)	106-122 (48-55.3kg)
5' 0" (152.4cm)	96-104 (43.5-47kg)	101-113 (45.8-51.2kg)	109-125 (49.4-56.6kg)
1" (154.9cm)	99-107 (44.8-48.5kg)	104-116 (47-52.6kg)	112-128 (50.7-58kg)

2" (158.5cm)	102-110 (46.2-49.8kg)	107-119 (48.5-53.9kg)	115-131 (52.1-59.4kg)
3" (160cm)	105-113 (47.6-51.2kg)	110-122 (49.8-53.3kg)	118-134 (53.5-60.7kg)
4" (162.6cm)	108-116 (48.9-52.6kg)	113-126 (51.2-57.1kg)	121-138 (54.8-62.5kg)
5" (165cm)	111-119 (50.3-53.9kg)	116-130 (52.6-58.9kg)	125-142 (56.6-64.3kg)
6" (167.6cm)	114-123 (51.7-55.7kg)	120-135 (54.4-61.2kg)	129-146 (58.5-66.2kg)
7" (170cm)	118-127 (53.5-57.5kg)	124-139 (56.2-63kg)	133-150 (60.3-68kg)
8" (172.7cm)	122-131 (53.3-59.4kg)	128-143 (58-64.8kg)	137-154 (62.1-69.8kg)
9" (175cm)	126-135 (57.1-61.2kg)	132-147 (59.8-66.7kg)	141-158 (63.9-71.6kg)
10" (177.8cm)	130-140 (58.9-63.4kg)	136-151 (61.6-68.4kg)	145-163 (65.7-73.9kg)
11" (180cm)	134-144 (60.7-65.3kg)	140-155 (63.4-70.2kg)	149-168 (67.5-76.1kg)
6'0" (182.8cm)	138-148 (62.5-67.1kg)	144-159 (65.3-72.1kg)	153-173 (69.3-78.4kg)

Note: Data is based on weights associated with the lowest mortality. To obtain weight for adults younger than 25 subtract 1 pound for each year under 25.

For ascertaining the height allow for a 1" heels for men and a 2" heels for women.

Calorie Table for Certain Common Foods and their usual combinations

Food	Calories	Added Item	Calories	Total Calories
Bread Whole-Wheat, 1 slice	**56**	Butter and Jam	**110**	**166**
Milk, skimmed 1 cup	**90**	Milk; whole 1 cup	**150**	**240**
Salad, Lettuce, and Tomatoes	**40**	Mayonnaise 1 tbs.	**100**	**140**
Peas 1 cup	**95**	Butter, 1tsp.	**60**	**155**
Potato, baked 1 avg., size	**95**	Butter, 1tbs.	**108**	**203**

Entrée	150	Gravy	100	250
Baked apple	90	Apple pie Homemade	320	410
	------		------	------
Total Calories	616		948	1564

Proper exercise is essential in any reducing programme. It doesn't necessarily have to include strenuous exercises like jogging, aerobics or swimming. Simply a brisk walk of 20 to 30 minutes thrice weekly will prove helpful and will increase the rate at which excess calories are burnt off. The following table will give you some idea of how quickly various sports or other activities burn off one hundred calories.

Minutes needed to use 100 calories during certain sports and other activities

Weight of Person

Activity	155lb.	130lb.
Skiing	8 mins.	9 mins.
Swimming at 2 m.p.h.	10 mins.	11 mins.
Running	11 mins.	13 mins.
Football	11 mins.	13 mins.
Tennis	14 mins.	17 mins.
Horseback riding	16 mins.	19 mins.

Gardening	17 mins.	21 mins.
Skating	19 mins.	23 mins.
Walking rapid	19 mins	23 mins.
Bicycling	24 mins.	29 mins.
Walking moderate, 3 m.p.h.	28 mins.	33 mins.
Golf	33 mins.	40 mins.

Exercise and Calorie Expenditure

Activity (for one hour)	**Calories**
Bicycling at 6 m.p.h.	240
Bicycling at 12 m.p.h.	410
Cross-country skiing	700
Jogging 5 m.p.h.	740
Jogging 7 m.p.h.	920
Jumping rope	750
Running in place	650
Running 10 m.p.h.	1280
Swimming 25 yards per minute	275
Swimming 50 yards per minute	500
Tennis singles	400
Walking 2 m.p.h.	240
Walking 3 m.p.h.	320
Walking 4 m.p.h.	440

From FDA consumer, July-August 1985

Here are some more suggestions on how to reduce and maintain your weight at an optimum level. Of course please remember that if you already have a chronic health problem you should always consult your physician before you take up any regime of dieting or exercise.

1. Do not be in a rush to reduce your weight. Slow and steady is the maxim you should follow and remember you should not loose more than two ponds a week.

2. Do not eat snacks between meals if you can help it.

3. Eat a good nutritious breakfast and lunch, but go easy on supper or dinner. Do not eat just before going to bed.

4. Learn to recognise the high calorie foods and avoid them.

5. Skip desserts; eat fresh fruit instead.

6. Avoid taking second helpings however much you are enjoying the food; always leave the table knowing that you could have eaten a little more.

7. Use lots of fruit, vegetables and whole grains. These will give you a feeling of fullness whilst at the same time keeping the calorie count down.
8. Cut down on fatty foods such as fatty meats, meat products, mayonnaise, salad dressing and nuts etc.

9. Purchase and learn how to use a calorie counter. Lower your calorie intake to a point where you are losing about 1 pound a week, but never more than two pounds. *Remember you loose weight by consuming fewer calories than you use.*

10. Establish a regular exercise programme that fits in easily with your needs, and stick to it.

Normal Diet For A Healthy Person

First observe the following rules for eating: —

Diet Rules

1. Do not eat fruit and vegetables together.
2. Do not eat between meals.

3. Do not drink any liquid with meals.
4. Allow five hours between meals.

Second, more care must be exercised in the cooking of food everyday so as not to destroy the vitamins, minerals and other life giving properties during preparation.

Third, 75 to 85 per cent alkaline food should be used in the everyday diet. If you have any ailments, your diet should be at least 90 per cent alkaline base forming foods. Eating acid foods brings on disease, while alkaline foods overcome disease and help to prevent it.

Fruits

all berries	apricots	apples	pears
grapefruit	cherries	lemons	plums
pineapple	raisins	grapes	figs
quinces	bananas	prunes	dates
peaches	oranges	melons	limes

Do not use cane sugar on fruits. Do not eat bananas unless they have dark spots on the skins and are not green at the ends. Dried fruits are good as long as they are not sulphured. Do not mix more than two kinds of fruit at a meal. It is best to eat fruit raw.

Vegetables

asparagus
beets
beet tops
celery
cabbage uncooked
cauliflower
carrots
cucumbers
turnips
tomatoes
dandelions
Irish potatoes unpeeled
kale
lettuce
onions
okra (lady finger)
parsley
all kinds of greens
watercress
parsnip
pumpkin (gourd)
rutabagas
sweet potatoes
squash
Swiss chard
all sprouts
spinach
beans

Legumes

soybeansgarbanzos (chickpeas)
green beans
dried beans of any kind
split peas
lentils
lima beans
peanuts
wax beans
navy beans
string beans
peas

Legumes are high in protein and therefore are useful as meat substitutes. As an example, peanut butter contains four grams of protein per tablespoon. The proteins contained in legumes are an adequate substitute for meat proteins if they are combined with proteins in wheat or corn products.

Approximate time require for Digestion (in hours)

Rice, boiled	1 hour
Barley, boiled	2 hours
Carrot boiled	3¼ hours
Beets, boiled	3½ hours
Egg (soft-boiled)	3 hours
Egg (hard-boiled)	3½ hours
Egg (fried)	3½ hours
Egg (raw)	2 hours
Butter	3½ hours
Bread, whole wheat	3½ hours
Bread, corn	3¼ hours
Vegetable, hashed warmed	2½ hours
Parsnips, boiled	2½ hours
Green corn and beans boiled	3¾ hours
Milk, boiled	2 hours
Milk, raw	2½ hours
Turnips, boiled	3½ hours

Potatoes, Irish (baked)	2½ hours
Potatoes, Irish (boiled)	3½ hours
Cabbage, raw	2½ hours
Cabbage, boiled	4½ hours
Apples, hard and sour, raw	3 hours
Apples, sweet and mellow, raw	2 hours

Essential Minerals

Macro-minerals		Micro-minerals
Calcium	Iron	Molybdenum
Phosphorous	Iodine	Chromium
Potassium	Zinc	Fluorine
Sulphur	Selenium	Silicon
Sodium	Manganese	Vanadium
Chlorine	Copper	Nickel
Magnesium	Cobalt	Tin

Going fashionably herbal may not always be the best thing. Stay safe by following these common sense guidelines prepared by the US Food and drugs Administration.

Garlic Capsules combined with diabetes medication can cause dangerous decrease in blood sugar. People sensitive to garlic may experience heartburn and flatulence. Garlic also has anti-clotting properties, so check with your doctor if you're on anti-coagulant drugs.

Ginseng the Korean wonder herb can increase blood pressure, so it's a no-no for those battling against hypertension. Steer clear if you've been prescribed a blood-thinning drug.

Gingko Biloba, the single most prescribed herbal medicine in the world, could have serious consequences (restlessness, nausea, diarrhoea and vomiting) for those taking drugs for high blood pressure or heart disease, or even aspirin.

Guarana, the much-advertised ingredient of energy drinks like Shock and Red Bull, contains 3-5 percent more caffeine than a cup of coffee. Avoid it if you've been advised by your doctor to stay away from caffeine. Long-term use may lead to decreased fertility, cardiovascular disease and many forms of cancer.

Kava Kava, another extremely popular herb with anti-anxiety, pain relieving, muscle relaxing and anti-convulsant effects, should not be used when you've had alcohol, sedatives or sleeping pills, or are on anti-psychotic drugs and medication for Parkinson's Disease.

Statutory Warning

One of the drawbacks of opting for patent over the counter herbal medicines especially without the guidance of qualified herbalists is that, "The absence of proper quality control mechanisms to verify the ingredients and the efficacy of drugs of alternative medicines has led to the proliferation of the practice of dispensing spurious drugs containing cortico-steroids" ***Dr. S K Gupta*** **Head of the Department of Pharmacology, All India Institute of Medical Science (AIIMS).**

Herbal Remedy Harms

They may be spiked with steroids
They may contain allopathic ingredients
They may have toxic metals
They may result in adverse reactions

They may react with allopathic drugs

One of the golden rules of using herbal medicine is never take any herb on a regular or long term basis without the advice of qualified practitioners. Always try to use fresh herbs and avoid patent medicines wherever possible. In fact it is better to identify, grow and preserve these herbs at home. Never use a herb unless you are absolutely sure of its credentials as a healing herb. This book is meant only as an introduction to the world of herbal medicine and the compiler and publisher can in no way take responsibility for any ill effects that may occur after using any of the remedies mentioned. If in doubt always consult a qualified practitioner before initiating any treatment with herbs.

Glossary of Medical Terms used

A

Abortifacient — An agent that promotes abortion.

Acne — A pimple-like eruption of the sebaceous glands of the skin, with accumulation of yellow secretion and black overgrowth of the horny layer of the skin.

After-pains — Painful contraction of the womb after childbirth.

Ague — An intermittent fever, sometimes with chills, as in malaria.

Alopecia — A disease of the scalp resulting in complete or partial baldness.

Alterative — A drug, which corrects disordered processes of nutrition and restores the normal function of an organ or system.

Amenorrhoea — Abnormal suppression of menses.

Anaemia — A deficiency of blood or red blood cells or of the red-colouring matter of the blood.

Analgesic — Any substance that relieves pain.

Anaphrodisiac — Herbs that decrease or allay sexual feelings or desires.

Anascara — Dropsy.

Angina pectoris— A disease of the heart marked by severe constricting pains in the chest.

Anodyne — A drug that relieves pain.

Antacid — A drug that neutralises acidity of the stomach.

Anthelmintic — A drug that kills intestinal worms.

Antibilious — A herb that combats biliousness. The term biliousness refers to a group of symptoms consisting of nausea, abdominal discomfort, headache, constipation and gas that is caused by an excessive excretion of bile.

Antibiotic	—	Inhibits the growth of germs, bacteria and harmful microbes.
Antiemetic	—	Prevents or alleviates nausea and vomiting.
Anti-epileptic	—	An agent that combats the convulsions or seizures of epile-psy.
Antihydrotic	—	A drug that checks sweating.
Antilithic	—	A drug that counteracts the development of stone or calculus.
Anti-periodic	—	Prevents the periodic recurrences of attacks of a disease; as in malaria.
Antiphlogistic	—	An agent that counteracts inflammation.
Antipyretic	—	Reduces fever. Same as febrifuge or Refrigerant.
Anti rheumatic	—	An agent that cures or relieves rheumatism.
Antiscorbutic	—	A drug that prevents or cures scurvy.
Antiseptic	—	Prevents decay or putrefaction. A substance that inhibits the growth and

development of microbes and microorganisms without necessarily destroying them.

Antispasmodic — A drug that counteracts spasmodic disorders.

Antisyphilitic — Herbs that cure or improve syphilis. Also called antiluetic.

Antitussive — Prevents or improves a cough.

Anti-venomous— Acts against poisonous matter from animals.

Anti-zymotic — Herbs that can destroy disease producing organisms.

Aperient — A mild purgative.

Aphrodisiac — A drug that promotes sexual desire.

Aphthae — Minute white ulcers on the tongue and in the mouth.

Apoplexy — Sudden loss of consciousness with some paralysis; stroke.

Ardor urine — A burning sensation on urinating.

Aromatic — A drug that is fragrant, spicy and mildly stimulant.

Ascaris — Intestinal parasitic roundworms.

Ascites — Abdominal dropsy.

Asthma — A chronic disorder of the bronchial tubes.

Astringent — A drug that arrests secretion or bleeding.

Atony — Lack of tension or muscular power.

Attenuent — An agent that dilutes fluids.

B

Balsam — The resin of a tree that is healing and soothing. For example myrrh.

Balsamic — A healing or soothing agent.

Bechic — A remedy for cough.

Bedsores — Ulceration of any part of the body of bedridden patient.

Beriberi — A deficiency disease caused by lack of vitamins especially B1.

Bitter — A solution of bitter, often aromatic, plant products used as mild tonic.

Black Smallpox— The hemorrhagic form of smallpox.

Blenorrhoea — Excessive mucous discharge, especially from the uro-genital organs.

Bright's disease— An acute or chronic disease of the kidneys.

Bronchitis — An inflammation of the air passages.

Bronchorroea — Excessive discharge from the bronchial mucous membrane.

C

Calculus — A hard and solid concretion formed in the body, especially in the urinary organs; it may be sand or gravel or stone, according to size.

Cancer — Any malignant grow-th.

Carbuncle — An acute suppurative inflammation of the skin and tissues under the skin, rapidly spreading around the original point of infection.

Caries — Decay of teeth.

Carminative — A drug that relieves flatulence.

Catarrh — The inflammation of the mucous membranes with free discharge. This has special reference to the air passages of the head and throat. For example, hay fever, rhinitis, influenza, bronchitis, pharyngitis and asthma.

Cathartic — A drug that induces active movement of the bowels.

Caustic — An agent that corrodes or destroys tissues.

Cephalic — Referring to diseases affecting the head and upper part of the body.

Cellulitis — Inflammation of the cellular tissues under the skin.

Chancre — A syphilitic ulcer.

Chilblains — Congestion of the blood at the extremities as a result of defective blood circulation caused by damp cold.

Cholagogue — A drug that promotes the flow of bile.

Cholera Infantum — A common, non-contagious diarrhoea seen in young children; occurs most commonly during the summer.

Cholera Morbus — A once popular name for an acute gastro-enteritis with diarrhoea, cramps, and vomiting occurring in the summer or autumn. Also called summer cholera or summer complaint.

Chorea — A disease chiefly of children, marked by irregular, spasmodic and involuntary actions of the limbs and face; St. Vitus's dance.

Chylous urine — Urine with a white milky fluid in which fat globules are in suspension.

Colic — Pain due to spasmodic contraction of the abdomen.

Condiment — Enhances flavour of food.

Congestion — An abnormal collection of blood in the blood vessels of any organ or part of the body.

Conjunctivitis — Inflammation of the conjunctiva, the mucous membrane covering the eyeball and lining the eyelids.

Contusion — An injury to the soft parts without breaking the skin.

Counterirritant— An agent that induces a mild irritation or inflammation of the skin to relieve congestion of the deeper structures.

Cordial — A stimulating medicine or drink.

Croup — A diseased condition of the larynx of children characterised by difficult and noisy breathing accompanied by a hoarse cough.

Cystitis — Inflammation of the bladder.

D

Dandruff — An inflamed condition of the scalp characterised by the presence of white scales in the hair due to the exfoliation of the horny cells of the scalp.

Delirium — An extreme mental disturbance marked by excitement, restlessness and rapid succession of confused and unconnected ideas.

Demulcent — An agent having a soothing effect on the skin and mucous membranes.

Deobstruent — A drug that removes an obstruction to secretion or excretion by opening the natural passages or pores of the body.

Depilatory — An agent that removes or destroys hair.

Depurative — Tends to purify and cleanse the blood.

Detergent — An agent that cleanses boils, ulcers and wounds etc.

Diabetes — A wasting disease of metabolism; in one form of the disease abundant sugar is present continuously in the urine; in the other form abundant sugar is not present but there is excessive discharge of urine, which of low specific gravity and pale in colour. Increase in blood sugar level. Diabetes is caused by the impaired secretion of insulin in the body.

Diaphoretic — A drug that induces copious perspiration.

Diphtheria — An infectious disease of the throat and the air passage, which become inflamed and swollen and are coated with a fibrinous exudate.

Discutient — A drug that disperses or absorbs a tumour or any coagulated fluid in the body.

Diuretic — A drug that increases the secretion and discharge of urine.

Drastic — A violent purgative.

Dropsy — A disease marked by an excessive collection of a watery fluid in the tissues or cavities of the body.

Dysentery — An infectious disease of which the chief symptoms are acute diarrhoea and discharge of mucous and blood.

Dysmenorrhoea — Usually painful and difficult menstruation.

Dyspepsia — Indigestion.

Dysuria — Painful and difficult urination.

E

Ecbolic	—	See Abortifacient.
Eczema	—	A skin disease accompanied by swelling, redness and exudation of lymph.
Elephantiasis	—	A disease of the skin caused by a tiny worm and attended with hypertrophy of the affected parts.
Emetic	—	A drug that induces vomiting.
Emmenagogue	—	A drug that promotes menstruation or regulates the menstrual periods.
Emollient	—	A drug that allays irritation of the skin and alleviates swelling and pain.
Enteritis	—	Inflammation of the intestines.
Epilepsy	—	A chronic nervous disorder marked by attacks of unconsciousness or convulsions.
Escharotic	—	An agent capable of destroying tissues.

Esculent — Edible or fit for eating.

Exanthematous— Refers to any eruptive disease or fever. A herbal remedy for skin eruptions such as measles, and scarlet fever etc.

Excoriation — Removal of skin by rubbing or chaffing.

Expectorant — A drug that promotes the removal of catarrhal matter and phlegm from the bronchial tubes; alleviates coughing.

F

Farinaceous — Of the nature of flour or meal. Starchy or containing starch.

Febrifuge — An agent for reducing fever.

Fistula — An abnormal channel that connects one cavity of the body with another, or which opens out from a cavity to the surface of the body.

Flatulence — A disorder in which there is an excessive collection of gas in the stomach.

Flux — Excessive flow or discharge. For example in dysentery or excessive menstruation.

Freckles — Coloured spots on the exposed parts of the skin.

G

Galactogogue — An agent that promotes the excretion and the flow of milk.

Gleet — A chronic discharge from the urethra either of mucus or pus; commonly seen in the chronic form of gonorrheal urethritis.

Glycosuria — A diseased condition of the urine in which sugar is excreted.

Goitre — A chronic enlarge-ment of the thyroid gland.

Gonorrhoea — An infectious vener-eal disease marked by an inflammatory discharge from the genital organs.

Gravel — A collection of tiny stone-like particles of uric acid, calcium oxalate or phosphates in the organs of the urinary system.

Griping — Sharp pain due to the presence of some irritating substance in the bowels.

Guinea worm — A very slender worm infecting human beings through drinking contaminated water; it gradually works its way into the subcutaneous tissues.

H

Haemoptysis — Spitting of blood from the lungs or bronchial tubes.

Haemorrhage — Bleeding especially profuse from any part of the body.

Heartburn — A burning feeling in the region of the chest and

		stomach, generally due to indigestion.
Hemicrania	—	Migraine.
Hemiplegia	—	Paralysis of one side of the body.
Hepatic	—	Pertaining to liver.
Hepatitis	—	Inflammation of the liver.
Hernia	—	Rupture; protrusion through its covering of any organ of the body.
Herpes	—	A deep-seated vesicular eruption causing neuralgic pains.
Hypnotic	—	A drug that induces sleep.
Hydragogue	—	A drug that causes discharge of watery fluid.
Hydrophobia	—	Rabies.
Hypochondriasis	—	A mental disorder in which the patient is tormented by melancholy views, particularly about his health.
Hysteria	—	A disease in which a physically healthy patient has lost control over acts and feelings and suffers from imaginary ailments.

I

Indolent	—	Painless; inactive.
Induration	—	Area of hardened tissue.
Intermittent fever	—	Fever that is marked by intervals of normal temperature between periods of rise of temperature.
Itch	—	An infectious skin disease, caused by a mite, without specific lesions and marked by excessive itching; scabies.

J

Jaundice	—	A diseased condition in which there is a yellowish staining of the tissues and excretions with bile.

L

Lactagogue	—	See Galactagogue.
Lactifuge	—	A drug that checks secretion of milk.

Laryngitis	—	Inflammation of the larynx.
Laxative	—	A herb that acts to promote the evacuation of the bowels; a gentle cathartic.
Leprosy	—	A chronic wasting disease caused by a germ; the disease generally results in mutilations and deformities.
Leucorrhoea	—	A whitish, viscid discharge from the vagina.
Leucoderma	—	A condition of the skin in which there is loss of pigment wholly or partially.
Lithotriptic	—	A drug used for removing calculi or stones formed in the urinary system.
Lochia	—	The vaginal discharge following childbirth.
Lochiorrhoea	—	Excessive flow of lochia.
Lumbago	—	Rheumatism of the muscles of the small of the back.
Lung Fever	—	A severe lung infection, as pneumonia.

M

Malaria — A recurrent disease marked by bouts of shivering, sudden rise of temperature and general aching of the body, ague.

Mania — A mental disorder marked by dangerous excitement or insane or morbid craving.

Maturating — An agent that promotes the maturing or bringing to a head of boils and carbuncles etc.

Measles — An infectious febrile disease, chiefly of children, marked by a cold in the head, running of the eyes and nose and appearance of tiny spots on the inner side of the cheek and of rash over the body.

Melancholia — A disorder of the mind marked by depression of spirits and mental sluggishness.

Menopause	—	Change of life.
Menorrhagia	—	Abnormally excessive menstruation.
Metrorrhagia	—	Bleeding from the womb.
Micturation	—	Urination.
Migraine	—	Periodic attack of headache affecting one side of the head.
Mortification	—	Gangrene.
Mucilaginous	—	Herbs that have a soothing effect on inflamed mucous membranes
Mumps	—	An infectious disease marked by the inflammation of the glands near the ear.

N

Narcotic	—	An addicting substance and drug that reduces pain and induces sleep.
Nausea	—	A feeling that vomiting is about to take place.
Nauseant	—	A herb that causes nausea and vomiting. Somewhat similar to an emetic.

Nephritis — Inflammation of the kidneys.

Nervine — A substance that calms and soothes the nerves and reduces tension and anxiety.

Neuralgia — Pain felt along a nerve.

Night-blindness — A disease in which the patient is incapable of seeing in the dark.

Nocturnal pollution — Involuntary discharge of the seminal fluid during the night.

O

Opthalmia — Conjunctivitis.

Opthalmicum — A remedy for diseases of the eyes.

Orchitis — Inflammation of the testicles.

Otitis — Inflammation of the ear.

Otorrhoea — A purulent discharge from the ear.

Ovaritis — Inflammation of the ovaries.

P

Parturient	—	A substance that induces and promotes labour.
Pectoral	—	A drug to cure disorders of the chest.
Peristalsis	—	Contraction and expansion of the intestines.
Pharyngitis	—	Inflammation of the pharynx.
Phythisis	—	Consumption; tuberculosis of the lungs.
Piles	—	An inflamed condition of the veins in the rectal region.
Pityriasis	—	A scaly skin disease.
Pleurisy	—	Inflammation of the membrane enclosing the lungs.
Pneumonia	—	Inflammation of the lungs.
Poultice	—	Plant material that is prepared in a special way and applied to the surface of the body as a remedy for certain disorders.

Prolapse — The falling downward of an organ of the body from its normal position.

Prophylactic — An agent that prevents disease.

Prurigo — A chronic skin disease marked by the eruption of small, rounded, reddish pimples.

Psoriasis — A common chronic inflammation of the skin, marked by rounded reddened patches that are covered with dry silvery scales.

Puerperium — The period between childbirth and the return of the womb to its normal condition.

Pulmonary — Pertaining to the lungs.

Pungent — Irritating or sharply painful. Producing a sharp sensation of taste or smell.

Purgative — A substance that promotes the vigorous evacuation of the bowels.

Usually used to relieve severe constipation.

Pyorrhea — A disease marked by purulent discharge from the gums.

Q

Quicksilver — An old term for mercury.

Quinsy — Peritonsillar abscess, or tonsillitis.

R

Refrigerant — A drug that relieves feverishness or produces a feeling of coolness.

Remittent fever— Fever in which the temperature fluctuates considerably, but does not drop to normal.

Relaxant — Tends to relax and relieve tension, especially muscular tension.

Resolvent — Promotes the resolving and removing of abnormal growths, such as tumour.

Rheumatism — An indefinite term used for pains in the muscles, joints and certain tissues.

Ringworm — A parasitic skin disease usually marked by red scaly, circular patches.

Roundworm — A pinkish intestinal, parasitic worm resembling the common earth worm.

Rubefacient — A mild counter irritant.

S

Scabies — An itching skin disease caused by a mite.

Scald Head — Ringworm, or some similar affliction, of the scalp. May also refer to a disease of the hair follicles with formation of small yellow crusts and a very offensive odour; usually affects the scalp.

Sciatica — An inflammation of the sciatic nerve at the back of the thigh.

Scorbutic — Suffering from scurvy.

Scrofula — Tuberculosis involving the lymph nodes of the neck, usually occurs early in life. Now very rarely seen.

Scurvy — A deficiency disease caused by the lack of vitamin

C.

Sedative — A drug that reduces excitement, irritation and pain.

Sialagogue — A drug that promotes salivation.

Sinus — Medically the term means a suppurating tract that has not healed up.

Sleeping Disease— Sleeping sickness; commonly found in Africa. Also viral encephalitis in which lethargy is a prominent feature.

Soporific — A drug that induces sleep.

Sprue — Chronic inflammation of the digestive tract, marked by indigestion and morning diarrhoea.

Stimulant — A herb that increases the activity or efficiency of a system or organ; acts more rapidly than a tonic.

Stomachic — Herbs that give strength and tone to the stomach, stimulate digestion, and improve the appetite.

Stomatitis — Inflammation of the mouth.

Strangury — Painful drop-by-drop discharge of urine.

Styptic — An agent that checks bleeding.

Sudorific — Herbs that cause heavy perspiration.

Summer complaint — See Cholera Morbus.

Syphilis — A chronic venereal disease.

T

Tenesmus — Involuntary, painful, spasmodic and frequent

straining to evacuate the bowels.

Tetanus — An infectious disease, marked by painful contraction in the muscles.

Tetters — A once popular name for various eczematous skin diseases. May also refer to a skin disease of animals communicable to man with intense itching.

Threadworm — A very small thin worm commonly infecting children, its habitat is in the large intestine.

Tincture — A solution of the active principle of a herb in alcohol.

Tonic — Herbs that restore and strengthen the entire system. Produces and restores normal tone. A general tonic would be one that braces up the whole system, such as a cold bath.

Tonsillitis — Inflammation of the tonsils.

Tympanitis — Distention of the abdomen due to the collection of gas.

Typhoid fever — An acute infectious disease characterised by ulceration of the intestines, eruption of rose coloured spots, and a typical course of temperature.

Typhus fever — An acute contagious and infectious disease marked by high temperature, and acute depression and eruptions.

U

Ulcer — An open sore on the skin.

Urethritis — Inflammation of the urethra, the can that extends from the bladder and discharges the urine.

Urticaria — An allergic disease of systemic origin marked by painful itching elevations of the skin.

V

Vermifuge — A drug that expels intestinal worms.

Vertigo — Dizziness.

Vesicant — An agent that produces a blister.

Vulnerary — A drug that promotes the healing of wounds.

W

Wart — A hypertrophy of or growth on the skin.

Whipworm — A common parasite in men; the worm has a thick body and a slender neck; it resembles a whip.

Whites — See Leucorrhoea.

Whitlow — A septic inflammation of the tissues surrounding the nail or the bone of the distal joint of a finger or toe.

Whooping cough— An acute infectious disease characterised by peculiar spasmodic attacks of coughing.

Z

Zymotic — Caused by or pertaining to any infectious or contagious disease.